10 Herbs for Happy, Healthy Cats

Lura Rogers

CONTENTS

Introduction

Centuries before veterinarians existed, cats in the wild instinctively relied on the medicinal powers of plants for healing. They were drawn to specific plants and their leaves, flowers, stems, and roots to cure a wide range of ills and aches, cuts and scrapes.

Today, our domesticated felines are living longer, healthier lives than their ancient ancestors, thanks in part to advances in traditional veterinary medicine. But as veterinarians and cat owners learn more about the benefits of holistic medicine, feline health care is increasingly returning to its plant-based roots. Veterinarians around the world are beginning to recognize the value of integrated medicine (combining traditional treatments with alternative ones such as herbs, acupuncture, and homeopathy). Membership in the American Holistic Veterinary Medical Association (see page 32 for the source of a directory) continues to grow each year as more veterinarians become trained in alternative medicine therapies.

Mother Nature's green pharmacy offers hundreds of herbs that can be helpful for felines. The "top 10" herbs profiled in this bulletin earn this acclaim because they are safe to use, are easy to obtain and administer, and address a wide range of common health conditions affecting our feline friends. When used properly, these herbs deliver a bounty of healing goodness, often free of the unpleasant side effects commonly associated with conventional medical prescriptions.

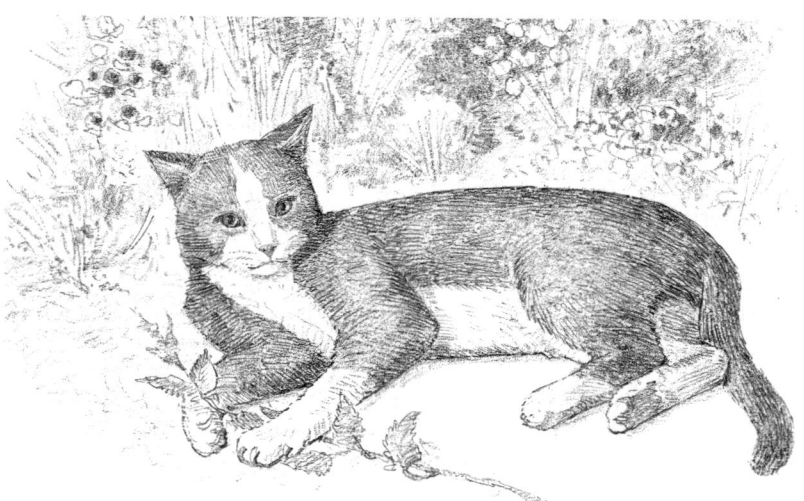

Plant medicines can contribute greatly to your cat's ongoing good health.

They not only treat symptoms but also, and more importantly, often enhance your cat's immune system and address the causes underlying health conditions.

You can buy these herbs in bulk or as tinctures, capsules, and salves from herb shops and natural foods stores. If you're a gardening enthusiast, however, you may want to grow your own, and you'll find the information you need here.

Ready to *purr*-sue this healing journey for you and your cat? Let's begin!

Using Herbs Safely

The herbal remedies suggested in this bulletin are safe and effective; if any precautions are advisable, I've noted them with each herb profile. However, there are a few general safety rules you should abide by:

- If your cat is taking any prescription medicine, I encourage you to seek the advice of a holistic-oriented veterinarian before supplementing with herbal remedies, because herbs and drugs can have harmful interactions.
- If you decide to branch out from the relatively safe and gentle herbs discussed here, you should seek the advice of a qualified professional before giving these new herbs to your cat.
- If you are using a commercial pet preparation, always follow label directions.
- More is not better. Some herbs offer potent benefits in small doses but in larger doses can be harmful. Always follow dosage instructions.
- Consult with your veterinarian before giving herbs to kittens or to pregnant or nursing cats. Their ever-changing physiology may not be able to safely handle doses of nature's medicine.
- Remember that some herbs work best when given regularly, while others are most effective when given on an as-needed basis. Read the herb profiles beginning on page 11, or consult with a holistic veterinarian or an herbalist for advice on how herbs can best be used for your cat.

Herbal Remedies — and Convincing Your Cat to Take Them

Most cat owners would gladly clean not one but a dozen litter boxes a day rather than attempt to give their cats medicine. I swear cats are psychic. They know what you have in mind before you even reach for the medicine bottle and dash under the bed or some other hiding spot. And even when you do catch them, they contour their bodies and make giving a pill, applying a salve, or administering eardrops a truly unpleasant event for all.

Let me share a little secret on how to outfox your cat. Never attempt to give your cat its medicine in an open area, like the kitchen or living room. The cat has too many escape routes. Instead, corner your cat in a small room, like the bathroom. Shut the door. Speak calmly but confidently. If you have a wiggly cat, wrap it gently in a big bath

---

Herbal Shopping Tips

There was a time when "shopping" for herbs was as simple as a walk in the woods. You simply grabbed a handful of whatever you needed. But those handfuls have become teas, tinctures, capsules, and other commercial preparations in a mind-boggling array of choices. If you want to make a smart buy, use these pointers as a checklist for your next herb purchase:

- Purchase products that list both the common name (such as valerian) and the scientific name (*Valeriana officinalis*) of each herb used. Proper identification is important because different plants often go by the same common name.
- Check for an expiration date.
- Choose products that give dosage instructions. Keep in mind that dosages are typically based on an average adult person weighing 150 pounds. Check with your vet to select the proper dosage for your cat.
- Whenever possible, buy only products with certified organic ingredients.
- Limit your purchases to one or two herbs or herbal products. Working with your holistic vet or an herbalist, take the time to see how effective these herbs are for your cat before trying other herbs.

---

towel, leaving only its head exposed. Once a cat realizes that there is no escape, it will wave the white flag of surrender. Always finish medicine-giving ordeals with lots of praise and a tasty treat. Then, open the door and let your cat scoot or saunter out, depending on its mood.

There are many herbal remedies available in the marketplace; most are high-quality products that you can feel comfortable buying and giving to your beloved pet. (See the box at left for tips on buying herbs and herbal products.) But if you're willing to commit the time, you can make your own herbal remedies at home — saving yourself some money, allowing you to customize blends for your cat's needs, and guaranteeing the quality of the preparation.

Fresh and Dried Herbs

Depending on the herb, you can use its flowers, leaves, stems, or roots in fresh or dried form; see the herb profiles beginning on page 11 for specifics on each plant. If you're growing your own herbs, you can snip fresh cuttings whenever you need them or harvest and dry the herbs for later use. You can also purchase dried herbs in bulk from herb shops and most natural foods stores.

To use fresh or dried herbs, chop them finely and mix them into your cat's food.

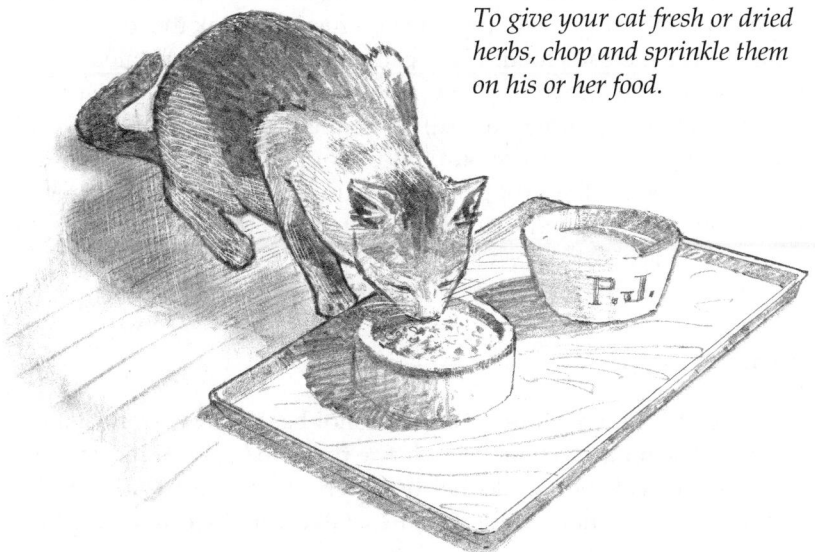

To give your cat fresh or dried herbs, chop and sprinkle them on his or her food.

Herbal Teas

Herbal teas are prepared by two main methods: infusion and decoction. To make an infusion, the herb is steeped. To make a decoction, the herb is simmered over time. Which technique you use depends on the type of herb you've selected.

Infusions. To extract medicinal properties from leaves, flowers, berries, or ground seeds, you infuse them. These ingredients easily release their essential oils when they're steeped in hot water — and they easily lose their value when they're simmered. To infuse a cup of tea, pour 1 cup boiling water over 1 to 2 teaspoons dried herbs or 2 to 4 tablespoons fresh herbs. Cover, let steep 10 to 15 minutes, and strain.

Decoctions. When the recipe calls for tougher herb parts — barks, roots, dried berries, seeds, or rhizomes — you need to use a brewing process known as a decoction. The simmering is necessary to extract the herb's valuable properties. To decoct a cup of tea, add 2 teaspoons dried root to 1 cup water. Cover, bring to a boil, simmer 15 to 20 minutes, and then strain.

Combinations. When you're making a tea with roots *and* leaves, you both infuse and decoct: Simmer the roots 20 minutes, remove the pot from the heat, add the leaves and stir, then cover and steep 10 to 20 minutes.

Note: Let the tea cool completely before giving it to your cat. Store any leftover tea in the refrigerator, where it will keep for up to 3 days.

Some cats will sweetly sip a cup of herbal tea if it contains the healing compounds they need. If your cat refuses to drink the tea, you can pour it over the cat's food. If the cat won't eat "contaminated" food, pour the dosage into a plastic syringe (available from your veterinarian or a veterinary supply house). Hold the cat's head with one hand, applying light upward pressure on the upper jaw with your thumb and fingers. Place the dropper in the side of your cat's mouth where the cheek pouch is, and deliver the herbal liquid in small but steady amounts. This pace makes your cat swallow each time.

Tinctures

Tinctures for humans are usually alcohol based. However, cats can have trouble metabolizing alcohol. The preferred solvent for tinctures intended for cats is not alcohol but glycerin, a sweet-tasting liquid available in most natural foods stores. Glycerin-based tinctures (also

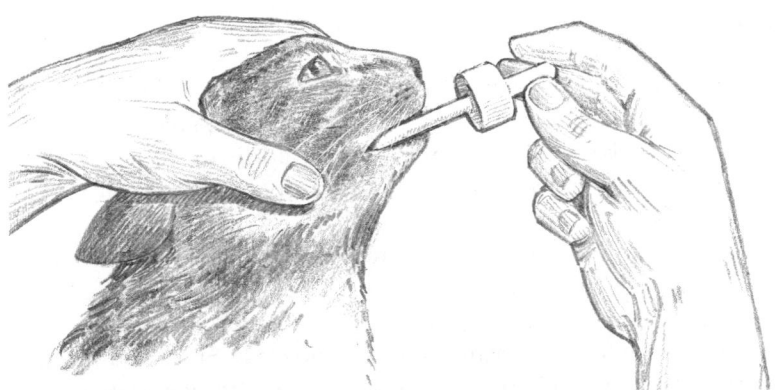

To give your cat liquid medicine, such as a tincture or tea, hold the cat's head securely and squirt the liquid from a plastic syringe into the cat's mouth.

known as glycerites) aren't as potent as alcohol-based tinctures and have a shorter shelf life (1 to 2 years). However, they are nonalcoholic. Glycerites are taken in small amounts — dropperfuls or teaspoonfuls.

There are many good glycerites available commercially. However, if you want to make your own, just follow these steps:

Step 1. Process the herbs. When you're using fresh herbs, coarsely chop or mince them. When using dried herbs, powder them in a coffee grinder or mortar and pestle.

Step 2. Put the processed herbs in a wide-mouthed jar. The herbs should make up about one-quarter of the total volume in the jar. Cover them with liquid. For fresh herbs, use twice as much glycerin as herb; for dried herbs, use three times as much glycerin as herb. Blend well.

Step 3. Seal the jar. Seal the jar tightly. Put the jar in a dark place, and let it sit for 3 to 6 weeks, shaking occasionally.

> ## Tincturing Tip
>
> If using glycerin and dried herbs, dilute the glycerin with ½ part water per part of glycerin. Use the glycerin at full strength when using fresh herbs.

Step 4. Strain and bottle the liquid. Strain the liquid and decant into smaller bottles, preferably made of dark glass. Store away from direct heat and light.

A tincture can be given like an herbal tea, either by mixing it into the cat's food or by administering with a plastic syringe.

Capsules

These supplements are a handy way for your cat to benefit from herbs without too much effort on a daily basis. Capsules are handy if your cat snubs food with any foreign additives but tolerates taking pills. Most herb shops and natural foods stores sell herbal capsules.

You can also custom-blend capsules to fit your cat's needs. Buy some small, empty pull-apart capsules at your local health food store. Use a clean coffee grinder or mortar and pestle to reduce the herbs to a fine powder. Fill each capsule halfway, and close. Since you will not want to do this on a daily basis, be sure to store extras in a well-sealed, dark-colored glass jar, preferably in the refrigerator or freezer.

The quickest method of administering a capsule is to insert the pill into a ball of moist cat food and serve it as a treat. Be sure to follow this up with another soft treat to make sure that your cat swallowed the pill.

If your cat keeps spitting out the pill, here's another option: Hold the cat's head with one hand, applying light upward pressure on the upper jaw with your thumb and fingers. Use your other hand to open the cat's mouth and pop the pill on its tongue as far back as possible. Then hold the cat's jaws closed and massage its throat to induce swallowing. Try blowing a quick puff of air into its face. When the cat blinks, he swallows — it's an automatic reflex (similar to the way we close our eyes when we sneeze).

Poultices

A poultice is a warm, moist mass of powdered or macerated fresh herb that is applied directly to your cat's skin to relieve insect bites and stings, inflammation, and blood poisoning. It works by drawing out infection, toxins, and foreign bodies embedded in the skin.

Poultices should be made only from herbs that are nontoxic. Your cat will most likely lick off the poultice preparation within an hour of its application. If you've used nontoxic herbs, this is not a problem. In fact, your cat licking off the poultice can contribute to the healing process by getting the herbs into the cat, where they can work internally to promote healing.

A poultice works best if it's prepared from fresh plant parts, but you can use dried herbs if that is what's available. Mash or grind the

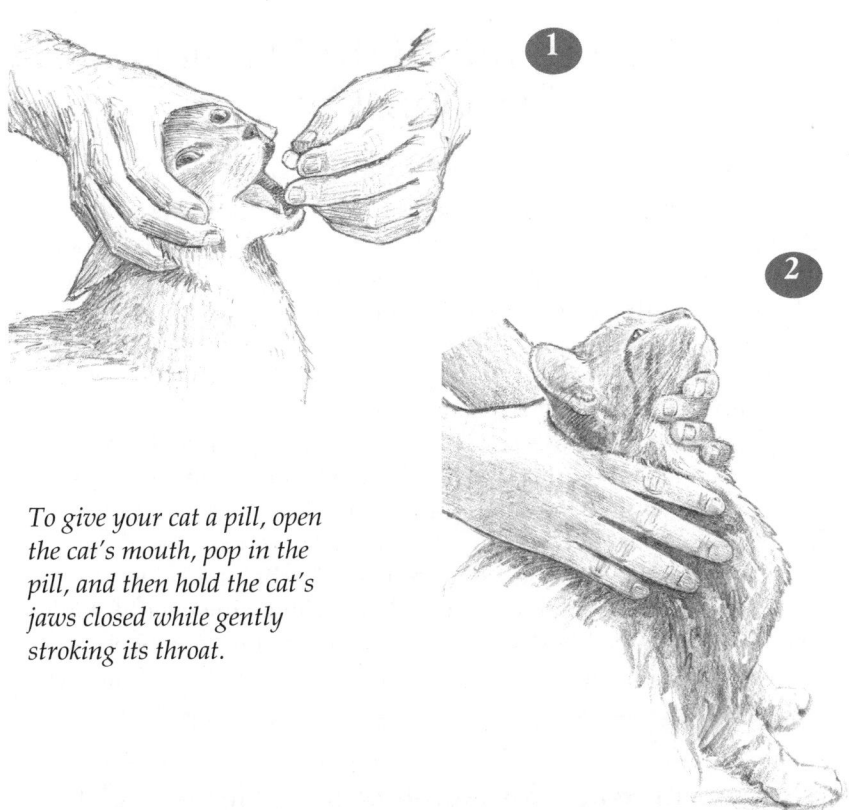

To give your cat a pill, open the cat's mouth, pop in the pill, and then hold the cat's jaws closed while gently stroking its throat.

herb, then mix with just enough boiling water to make a thick paste. Allow to cool to room temperature, then apply directly to the spot that needs attention.

Change the poultice frequently if the wound is bad; less frequently if it is minor. Generally, poultices should be kept in place for an hour, but the time varies with the herb and the severity of the condition.

If your cat keeps licking off the poultice as soon as it's applied, consider getting an Elizabethan collar (a plastic funnel-shaped collar that fits around the cat's neck) from your veterinarian or a pet supply store. Have your cat wear this collar for an hour or so after you apply the poultice. An Elizabethan collar will prevent a cat from licking off a poultice, but it won't prevent the cat from scratching off the poultice. If your cat is particularly determined not to have that poultice and manages to keep scratching it off even while wearing the Elizabethan collar, you may have to bow to its wishes.

Finding the Right Dosage for Your Cat

The easiest and safest way to give herbal dosages is to give them to effect. The basic rule is to start out slowly, with low doses at first. Then, after a month or so, when the cat adjusts to her herbal intake, taper off or add on, depending on her reaction. Often very small amounts of herb are enough to activate a cure.

Expect slow and easy results. Herbs most often need to be given for at least 30 days before you'll see appreciable results. Look for mild and subtle — and long-lasting — changes.

There are many different delivery systems for herbal remedies, some of which are outlined below. Use whichever one is easiest to give to your cat. It is more important to get the herbs into the cat's system than it is to worry about the "proper" way to dose them.

As a general rule, you can administer herbal medicine to your cat following the guidelines in the chart below. However, if you're using a commercial herbal remedy, always follow the label directions, because dosages can vary among different herbs and different herbal forms.

General Rules for Administering Herbs to Cats

Adapted from *Dr. Kidd's Guide to Herbal Cat Care*,
by Randy Kidd, D.V.M. (Storey Books, 2000)

Cat's Weight	Sprinkles (put on the cat's food once daily)	Teas (poured over food or into the cat's water)
1–5 lbs.	A very small pinch	⅛ cup once daily
5–10 lbs.	A small pinch	⅛ to ¼ cup one or two times daily
10–20 lbs.	A bigger pinch	¼ cup one or two times daily
Over 20 lbs.	2 pinches to 1 teaspoon	¼ to ⅓ cup one or two times daily

10 Herbs to Know

Without a doubt, catnip rules as felines' favorite herb. It adds zip and zest to our cats, providing us with lots of amusing antics to watch. Beyond catnip, it's easy to be confused about which botanicals to buy. With the dozens of herbs available, you could go broke trying to keep a supply of every one of them.

I'm here to save you time and money. My 10 favorite herbs for cats are easy to administer, offer varied and versatile healing benefits for common cat ailments, are safe to use, and are widely available. Here's the lineup:

- Burdock (*Arctium lappa*)
- Calendula (*Calendula officinalis*)
- Caraway (*Carum carvi*)
- Catnip (*Nepeta cataria*)
- Dill (*Anethum graveolens*)
- Echinacea (*Echinacea angustifolia, E. purpurea*)
- Eyebright (*Euphrasia officinalis*)
- Parsley (*Petroselinum crispum*)
- Rosemary (*Rosmarinus officinalis*)
- Valerian (*Valeriana officinalis*)

Capsules/Tablets (administered orally)	Tinctures (in the cat's water or food or given directly by mouth)
Small chip of a tablet or ⅛ to ¼ capsule 1 to 2 times daily	1 to 3 drops one to three times daily
¼ to ½ capsule or tablet one or two times daily	3 to 5 drops one to three times daily
½ to 1 capsule or tablet one to three times daily	3 to 5 drops one to three times daily
½ to 1 capsule or tablet two to four times daily	5 to 10 drops one to three times daily

Burdock
(Arctium lappa)

Parts used: Roots

Of historical note: Burdock root, also known as gobo, is considered a vegetable in Asian cultures. Burdock arrived on the North American continent with early European colonists. Burdock's infamous burrs inspired the creation of Velcro.

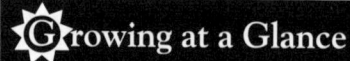

Growing at a Glance

PLANT CYCLE:
  Biennial

SOIL REQUIREMENTS:
  Prefers loam but will tolerate most soil conditions

LIGHT REQUIREMENTS:
  Full sun, partial shade, or shade

Medicinal uses: Burdock has incredible blood-cleansing capabilities and offers excellent support to the liver, urinary tract, and skin. By enhancing kidney function and cleansing the liver, it helps felines clear their systems of waste and toxins. It is especially helpful in easing the symptoms of arthritis and improving skin conditions.

The easiest method of giving burdock to your cat is to grind the root into a powder and sprinkle it on your cat's food. You can also give your cat burdock tea or tincture.

Growing your own: Because of its sticky burrs, not many gardeners enjoy having burdock around. But burdock root is harvested after its first year of growth, and in that first year, burdock produces only a rosette of leaves — no big plant, no flowers, no seeds, and no sticky burrs.

To grow this biennial herb, sow seeds in early spring. Burdock grows in just about any location; the plant prefers loam but tolerates most soil conditions. Burdock seeds germinate quickly, and seedlings should be thinned to about 18 inches apart.

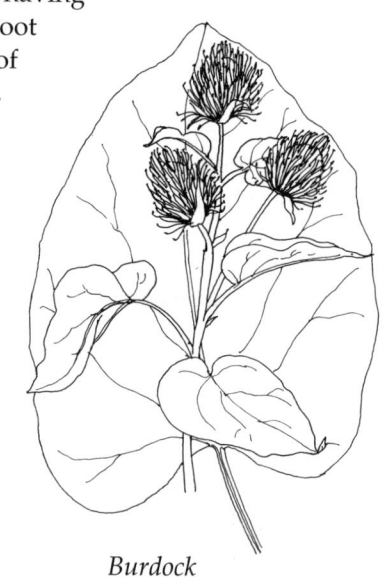

Burdock
(Arctium lappa)

Harvesting and storing: Harvest burdock's deep taproot in the fall of the first year or the spring of the second year.

Cautions: In rare cases, burdock leaves cause contact dermatitis. Some felines experience diarrhea with extended use of burdock; if this happens, simply stop giving the herb to your cat.

BURDOCK DAILY DETOX SUPPLEMENT

Adapted from *10 Herbs for Happy, Healthy Dogs,*
by Kathleen Brown (Storey Books, 2000)

This daily supplement will help clear your cat's system of toxins. Burdock, nettle, and red clover are great tonic herbs, supporting and strengthening the body's systems. Calendula aids in liver function and gives the immune system a boost.

> 1 teaspoon dried burdock root
> 2 cups water
> 1 teaspoon dried calendula blossoms
> 1 teaspoon dried nettle leaves
> 1 teaspoon dried red clover blossoms

To make a tea:
Add the burdock root to the water and bring to a boil. Reduce heat, cover, and let simmer 10 to 15 minutes. Remove from the heat, add the remaining herbs, and steep, covered, 10 minutes. Strain and allow the tea to cool.

To make capsules:
You can also make capsules with this formula, following the instructions on page 8.

To use:
Administer orally, following the dosage guidelines on page 11.

Calendula
(Calendula officinalis)

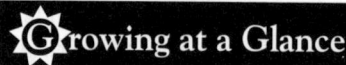

Parts used: Flowers

Of historical note: Calendula has been prized throughout history not only for its medicinal uses but also as a symbol of victory. Civil War soldiers and cowboys in the Wild West used calendula as a poultice to help heal bullet wounds.

Medicinal uses: Calendula's primary medicinal use is as a topical treatment for cuts and burns. It also

PLANT CYCLE:
Annual

PROPAGATION:
Seed

SOIL REQUIREMENTS:
Fertile, well-drained, pH 6.0–7.0

LIGHT REQUIREMENTS:
Full sun to partial shade

works to soothe the itching and irritation of insect bites, poison ivy and poison oak rashes, flea bites, and surgical incisions. Calendula poultices and salves are wonderful for helping to accelerate the healing of minor wounds, bruises, scratches, rashes, and sores. You can also use them on healing incisions to speed recovery.

Taken internally as a tea or tincture or in capsule form, calendula is antimicrobial and antiviral. It stimulates the immune system, calms the nervous system, and aids in liver function.

Growing your own: Also known as pot marigold, calendula is a sturdy annual that grows 12 to 15 inches high. The bright orange and yellow flowers bloom from early summer through autumn, closing up each evening and reopening in the morning. Deadhead throughout the season to encourage further blooming.

Calendula prefers full sun; it does well in just about any soil as long as it is well drained. The herb is easily started from seed. Sow directly in the ground in early spring, when the soil temperature has reached 60°F, or start indoors and transplant later. Space the plants 9 inches apart.

Harvesting and storing: Pluck the flowers in the afternoon, when they are just fully open. Place the flowers on paper towels in an area with good air circulation and out of direct sunlight.

Cautions: Calendula should not be used for pregnant cats. Do not use calendula on wounds that need to drain, such as abscesses; calendula is such a potent healer that it may cause the wound to heal too quickly, trapping the infection inside. Use only the flowers, as calendula leaves and stems contain minute amounts of salicylic acid, which is potentially toxic to cats.

FRESH CALENDULA OINTMENT

If you have calendula growing in your garden, you can make a fresh oint-
ment to speed the healing of minor cuts and scrapes.

> **Fresh calendula petals**
> **Olive oil**

To make:
Crush the fresh flowers with a mortar and pestle until they are
bruised and broken. Add just enough olive oil to create a paste,
mixing together well. You can refrigerate any unused portion (it
will keep for up to 3 days), but the ointment is most potent when
fresh.

To use:
Spread the ointment over your cat's scrape. Reapply as necessary.

CALENDULA PASTE

If you don't have fresh calendula for making an
ointment, try making this paste, which is also
excellent for helping feline cuts and scrapes
heal quickly.

> **1 part ground dried calendula petals**
> **1 part cornstarch or arrowroot**
>   **powder**
> **Spring water**

To make:
Mix together the calendula powder and
the cornstarch. Add just enough water
to create a thick paste. Store in a tightly
sealed container in the refrigerator, where
the paste will keep for up to 2 weeks.

To use:
Spread the paste over your cat's cut or
scrape. Reapply as necessary.

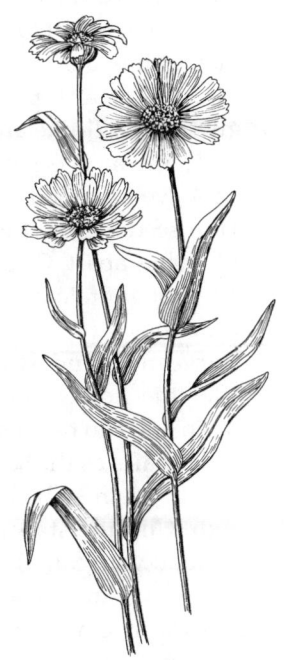

Calendula
(Calendula officinalis)

Caraway (Carum carvi)

Parts used: Seeds

Of historical note: In colonial times, parishioners often carried caraway seeds in small pouches to prayer meetings; they ate the seeds to curb their appetites and keep their stomachs from rumbling during silent prayers.

Medicinal benefits: Caraway seeds are well-known as kitchen seasonings, but they also help stimulate the appetite and ease occasional bouts of diarrhea and upset stomach. To use, grind or crush the seeds and sprinkle them on your cat's food.

Growing your own: Caraway is a biennial herb that grows to about 2 feet in height. During its first season the plant produces a rich display of foliage. The following spring new foliage appears, followed by a tall stem topped by an umbel of small white flowers, which give off a dill-like aroma.

Caraway is easily grown from seed. It prefers full sun and a dry, light, well-drained soil. Sow seeds about 2 weeks before the last frost. Thin seedlings so that they are between 6 and 12 inches apart. Once established, the plants are drought tolerant and don't need much watering.

Harvesting and storing: A few weeks after the flowers fade, the small seeds ripen and can be harvested. Harvest the aerial parts as the seeds turn brown. Be sure to get them before they fall on their own. Clip the stalks down far enough so that you can tie them together in bunches. Hang bunches upside down in a warm, dry area, placing a tray covered in paper underneath. After the seeds drop, allow them to dry completely for two weeks before storing them in tightly sealed containers.

Cautions: None.

Growing at a Glance

PLANT CYCLE:
Biennial, Zones 3–8

PROPAGATION:
Seed

SOIL REQUIREMENTS:
Well-drained, fertile, pH 6.0–7.0

LIGHT REQUIREMENTS:
Full sun

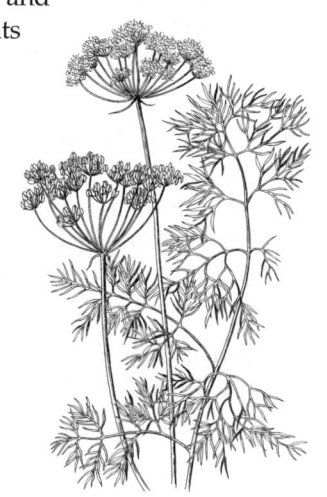

Caraway
(Carum carvi)

CARAWAY MILK FOR UPSET STOMACHS

Got a kitty with an upset tummy? Try this stomach-calming recipe. In fact, make a cup for yourself and set out the extra in a dish for your cat. Serve up this recipe only for periodic bouts of indigestion, because the lactose in milk is not good for cats in large quantities. If your cat is lactose intolerant, substitute water for milk and pour the tea over her food.

> 1–2 tablespoons caraway seeds
> 1 cup whole milk

To make:
Crush the seeds with a mortar and pestle. In a medium-sized saucepan, bring the milk to a boil, stirring frequently so that it doesn't scald. Turn off the heat and add the crushed seeds. Cover and let steep for 20 minutes, then strain out the seeds.

To use:
Give your cat a small dish of the milk, and add the softened seeds to her food.

Catnip (Nepeta cataria)

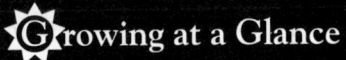

Growing at a Glance

PLANT CYCLE:
Perennial, Zones 4–9

PROPAGATION:
Seed, stem cuttings

SOIL REQUIREMENTS:
Sandy, well-drained, pH 7.0–8.0

LIGHT REQUIREMENTS:
Full sun to partial shade

Parts used: Aerial parts
Of historical note: Catnip has been a favorite of felines for centuries. Its genus name, *Nepeta*, derives from the ancient Roman town of Nepeti, where the herb grew wild in abundance. In those times, the herb was thought to symbolize happiness, love, and beauty.
Medicinal uses: Catnip's leaves, stems, and flowers are filled with compounds that work in harmony to relieve muscle spasms, colds, fevers, diarrhea, and gas in cats as well as people. In cats, catnip acts initially as a stimulant, then becomes sedative. Drawn by its scent, cats chew on the plant to release its active chemical, nepetalactone. Catnip is also an excellent herb for high-strung cats with nervous stomachs.

Give your cat fresh or dried crushed leaves or a glycerin-based catnip tincture. Some people have had success dropping a few leaves in their cats' water bowls.

Growing your own: A perennial member of the Mint family, catnip grows easily in the wild and is hardy in Zones 4 to 9. You'll have to fence off the catnip plants in your garden to prevent them from being conquered by neighborhood cats, or you'll simply have to plant enough catnip so there is plenty to go around. Whatever you do, don't put the catnip in the midst of fragile plants in your garden, or they will surely be flattened.

Plant catnip in full sun; the more sun the plants get, the more nepetalactone they produce. Sow seeds directly in the ground in early to midspring, or start indoors and transplant in late spring. You can also propagate catnip from stem cuttings (see the box below for instructions), which should be taken in spring or early summer and planted about 4 inches deep in soil. If you keep the soil around them moist, the cuttings should root within a week.

Harvesting and storing: Catnip should be harvested in late summer while it is in full bloom. The flowering tips of the plants are the most potent. Cut off the tops and leaves, or pull up the entire plant and

---

Taking a Cutting

Adapted from *Herbal Remedy Gardens,* by Dorie Byers (Storey Books, 1999)

Prepare clean containers and a light seed-starting mix. Straight vermiculite works well. With sharp scissors, cut 3 to 6 inches off the chosen stem just below a leaf node (where leaves emerge from the stem). Strip off the lower leaves, and remove any blooms from the cutting. If you are using rooting hormone, dip the stem into it. Insert the lower half of the cutting into the potting mix. Firm the mix around the stem, making sure there are no air pockets. Place the cutting in a warm spot out of direct light. Lightly mist with room-temperature water twice a day. Do not overwater; the soil should be kept damp but not waterlogged. Be patient. It will take several weeks for roots to form. You will know that the cuttings have taken root when a plant resists being pulled up with gentle tugging or there is new top growth.

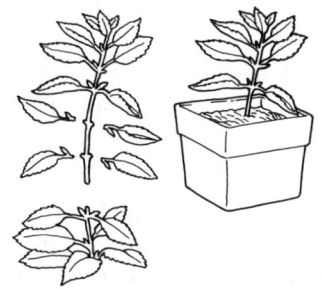

Strip the lower leaves from the cutting before inserting it into the potting mix.

hang it upside down to dry; either way, select a shady, dry area. Store the herb in an airtight container out of the sunlight — and out of your cat's reach.

Cautions: Wait until your cat is at least 6 months old before introducing it to catnip. Do not give catnip to pregnant cats.

Dill
(Anethum graveolens)

Parts used: Aerial parts
Of historical note: The name for this tall, elegant plant comes from the Norse *dilla,* which means "to lull."
Medicinal uses: Dill is generally used as a stomach-soothing agent for cats. It can help relieve nausea and flatulence, especially when triggered by a sudden change in diet. The seeds are most potent, but there is plenty of healthy goodness in the foliage and flowers. Feed your cat fresh or dried dill, or give it in tea or tincture form.

☀ Growing at a Glance

PLANT CYCLE:
Annual
PROPAGATION:
Seed
SOIL REQUIREMENTS:
Fertile, well-drained, pH 5.5–6.5
LIGHT REQUIREMENTS:
Full sun

Growing your own: Dill is an annual herb that features large umbels of small yellow flowers that bloom from mid- to late summer. The plant's long, thin stalks reach 3 feet in height and should be staked for support.

Dill prefers full sun and well-drained soil. Sow seeds directly in the ground in early spring, after the frosts have gone. Space the plants at least 8 inches apart.

Harvesting and storing: Seeds are best harvested about two to three weeks after the flowers blossom. Cut the stalks and hang them upside down over paper towels in a warm, dark location. The seeds will fall as they dry. Give the seeds another few days to dry completely before storing them in airtight containers.

Cautions: Do not give dill to pregnant or nursing cats, except under the supervision of your veterinarian.

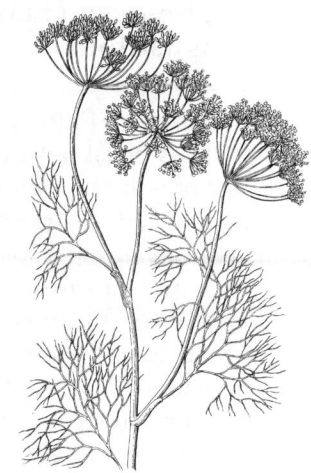

Dill (Anethum graveolens)

CARAWAY-DILL TUMMY-SOOTHING CAT SNACK

Try this herbal blend the next time your cat is suffering from stomach upset due to a change in diet.

    2 tablespoons caraway seed
    2 tablespoons dill seed
    1 tablespoon valerian root
    1 tablespoon dried rosemary
    1 tablespoon dried parsley
    1 6-ounce can tuna or chicken in water
    ¾ cup cooked rice
    3 tablespoons soy sauce

To make:
Combine the caraway seed, dill seed, valerian, rosemary, and parsley and grind in a mortar and pestle. Place the canned meat (including the water), rice, soy sauce, and herb mixture in a blender or food processor. Mix well, adding rice or water to adjust the consistency to your cat's liking. Store the unused portion in a tightly sealed container in the refrigerator, where it will keep for up to a week. You can also freeze individual servings to thaw as needed.

To use:
Feed your cat ¼ cup of the mixture per day.

Echinacea (Echinacea angustifolia; E. purpurea)

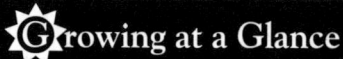

Growing at a Glance

PLANT CYCLE:
  Perennial, Zones 3–8

PROPAGATION:
  Seed, division

SOIL REQUIREMENTS:
  Well-drained, pH 5.5–7

LIGHT REQUIREMENTS:
  Full sun to partial shade

Parts used: Entire plant
Of historical note: Echinacea was a favorite herb in the medicinal arsenal of Native Americans, who were well aware of its potency. They used echinacea to treat everything from snakebites to burns.
Medicinal uses: Echinacea has tremendous benefits for the immune system, and it also works wonders for respiratory and skin conditions. Give your cat echinacea tea, echinacea tincture, or the fresh leaves, stems, and flowers. You can also apply echinacea as a poultice to relieve pain and swelling associated with insect bites and stings.

Growing your own: This easy-to-grow perennial produces lovely pink-purple flowers from mid- to late summer. *E. angustifolia* prefers poorer soil that is not overly moist, while *E. purpurea* prefers richer soil and regular watering; both species grow best in full sun.

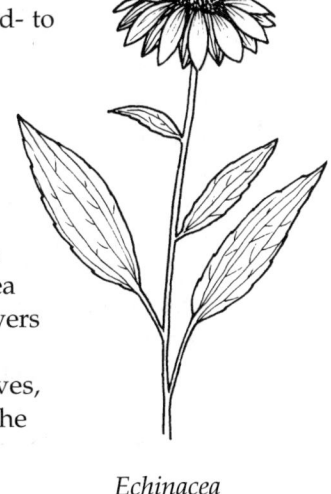

Echinacea is easily started from seed or by division (see the box on page 22). Echinacea seeds need to be stratified, so sow them in late fall. Space plants at least 1½ feet apart. Echinacea will reach a height of 1 to 2 feet, and the flowers should be deadheaded to prolong blooming.

Harvesting and storing: Aerial parts — leaves, flowers, and seeds — can be harvested after the plant's second year. Roots can be harvested in spring or autumn of the plant's third year. Allow echinacea to dry in a warm location away from direct sunlight and with plenty of air circulation. Once dried, store the herb

Echinacea
(Echinacea angustifolia)

in an airtight container. Do not pregrind the roots; leave them whole until you need them, to preserve their potency.

Cautions: Do not give echinacea to cats with abnormally functioning immune systems, such as cats diagnosed with diabetes or feline immunodeficiency virus (FIV), except under the advice of a qualified physician. In addition, note that many cats have a bad reaction to echinacea, including frothing at the mouth, crying, and hiding. Such reactions usually lessen in severity after the first-time dose.

ECHINACEA-CALENDULA HEALING POULTICE

This quick remedy is excellent for soothing the pain and inflammation of bee stings and minor burns.

> ¼ **cup fresh echinacea root**
> ¼ **cup fresh calendula leaves**
>   **Spring water**

To make:
Grind the echinacea and calendula. Add just enough warm water to create a paste.

To use:
Place a dollop of the paste on the wound. Change the dressing as needed.

Propagating Herbs by Division

Adapted from *Herbal Remedy Gardens,* by Dorie Byers (Storey Books, 1999)

Division is good not only for obtaining new plants but also for reviving perennials. The ideal time to divide is in spring. Lift the mother plant in its entirety from the ground with a garden fork. Shake the soil from the roots. Look at the plant for natural divisions. Each division should have some roots and one or two stems. Gently pull apart the plant or cut it cleanly with a knife. Water the divisions thoroughly, and trim some of the top growth. (Leaving too much top growth will cause new divisions to lose moisture.) Keep the new plantings well watered. Watch for new growth, a sign that the plants are established.

Eyebright (Euphrasia officinalis)

Parts used: Aerial parts

Of historical note: Eyebright derives its name from its long-time use as a remedy for eye ailments.

Medicinal uses: If your cat has an eye that is weepy, red, and irritated, eyebright — either taken internally as a tea or tincture or used externally as an eyewash — can help clear up the problem. When used internally and externally, eyebright can help treat herpesvirus infections, one of the most common eye infections in cats. As an anticatarrhal (mucus-clearing agent), anti-inflammatory, and astringent, eyebright is also helpful in treating upper respiratory disease. For best results, use eyebright in combination with immune-stimulating herbs such as echinacea and blood-cleansing herbs such as burdock.

Growing your own: Eyebright could be considered a robber baron of the plant world. This semiparasitic plant penetrates the roots of a host plant — commonly clover, plantain, or one of the many species of grasses — and absorbs from it the nutrients it needs to grow.

☀ Growing at a Glance

PLANT CYCLE:
Annual

PROPAGATION:
Seed

SOIL REQUIREMENTS:
Tolerates most soil conditions

LIGHT REQUIREMENTS:
Full sun to partial shade

This small annual is delicate in nature, with weedy overtones. The tiny red or white flowers sprout in abundance on thin stems that are scraggily appointed with small leaves.

Eyebright requires a wild area removed from your cultivated garden. Eyebright does not transplant well and should be sown directly. To propagate, simply over-seed a thin, grassy, moist area with eyebright seed in early spring.

Harvesting and storing: Gather the plant in late summer or early autumn while it is in bloom. Allow it to dry in a warm location away from direct sunlight and with plenty of air circulation. Once dried, store the herb in an opaque airtight container.

Cautions: None.

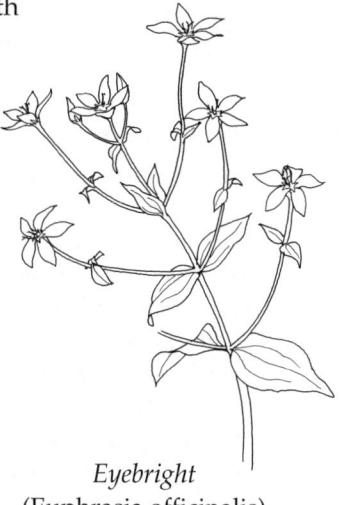

Eyebright
(Euphrasia officinalis)

EYEBRIGHT EYEWASH

This easy-to-make remedy helps ease irritation and clears up any discharge coming from the eye. Be sure to wash your hands before and after treatment. To compound the healing effects, also give your cat an infusion of eyebright (see instructions on page 6) internally.

> 2 cups water
> 1 teaspoon dried eyebright

To make:
Bring the water to a boil. Remove from heat and stir in the eyebright. Cover and let steep 10 minutes, then strain. Allow to cool to room temperature.

To use:
Using an eyedropper, drip 2 drops of the solution in each of your cat's eyes.

Caution

Eye irritations may signal that your cat has a foreign object trapped in the eye, a tear in the cornea, or a more serious infection. Before treating your cat at home, bring it to a veterinarian for a proper diagnosis.

Parsley
(Petroselinum crispum)

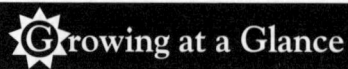
Parts used: Roots, leaves, and seeds

Of historical note: Ancient Romans wore parsley garlands around their necks at banquets in the hope that the herb would soak up wine fumes and keep them from getting drunk. Europeans during the Middle Ages wore parsley on Good Friday to ward off evil spirits.

Medicinal uses: One of parsley's greatest attributes is its high vitamin content. It is full of vitamins A, B-complex, and C, as well as iron, calcium, and potassium. The root, which is high in potassium, can be used as a diuretic, laxative, and eyewash. Eaten raw or taken as a tea or tincture, the leaves can help alleviate bladder problems and freshen breath.

Growing your own: Parsley does well in most soil conditions in full sun to partial shade. Parsley takes a long time to germinate (typically 6 weeks). To speed up the process, soak the seeds in water for 24 hours before sowing. Sow seeds directly into the ground in early spring, when the soil has reached 50°F. Water the seeds frequently to help speed germination. Thin plants to about 8 inches apart.

Harvesting and storing: Fresh parsley is much more potent than dried. Snip it as needed throughout the summer. To dry it, hang the plant, or lay the aerial parts on a screen in the shade. Crumble the dry leaves by hand and store in a well-sealed glass container.

Cautions: Do not give parsley to pregnant cats; use sparingly for nursing felines. Do not give parsley to cats diagnosed with kidney disease.

The Incredible Edible Herb

Because parsley is packed with nutrition, and because fresh parsley is so much more potent than dried, you may simply want to serve up your cat's meal with a parsley garnish. Parsley has a "green" taste that most cats enjoy, and your cat may eat it with no encouragement from you.

Rosemary
(Rosmarinus officinalis)

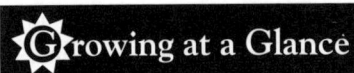

Parts used: Leaves, flowers, and stems
Of historical note: Rosemary has long been prized for its stimulating scent and pretty blue flowers. It is said that the flowers took on this beautiful hue when the Virgin Mary hung her legendary blue cloak on the branches of a rosemary bush. The ancient Greeks believed that wreaths of rosemary worn on the head would improve the function of the mind. Considered a symbol

PLANT CYCLE:
Tender perennial, Zones 8–10

PROPAGATION:
Stem cutting

SOIL REQUIREMENTS:
Well drained, pH 6.0–6.5

LIGHT REQUIREMENTS:
Full sun

of friendship and remembrance, rosemary garlands are often worn at weddings and funerals.

Medicinal uses: This versatile antioxidant herb repels insects, relieves flatulence, and eases muscular and nerve pain. It helps ease the itch and dryness associated with eczema and soothes the soreness of arthritis. You can apply a rosemary poultice or a cloth soaked in a strong rosemary tea on your cat's arthritic joints to draw blood from the area and ease the pain. You can also give rosemary tincture internally to help your cat relax, especially after a scary or traumatic experience.

Growing your own: Rosemary prefers full sun and well-drained soil. This herb is tough to start from seed. I recommend propagating rosemary from stem cuttings (see the box on page 18 for instructions), which should be treated with liquid rooting hormone. Keep the cuttings moist but not soggy until a strong root structure has formed.

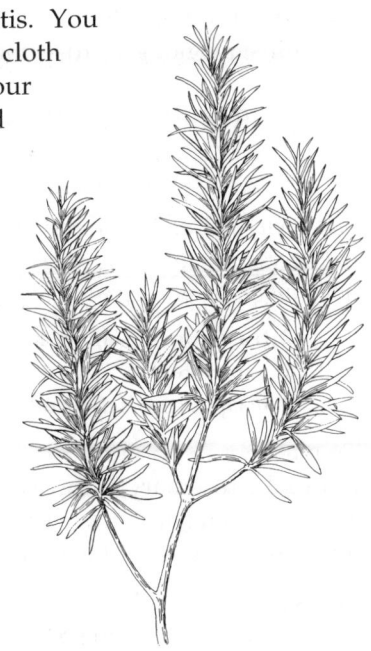

Rosemary
(Rosmarinus officinalis)

Because rosemary is a tender plant, it must be brought indoors for the winter in climates cooler than Zone 8. I recommend growing rosemary in pots in these cool-climate areas. You can bury the pots in your garden during the summer and then dig them out and bring them indoors for the winter. Of course, you can also grow rosemary indoors year-round.

Rosemary benefits from a soil "fluffing" each year, which keeps the soil from becoming too tightly packed and preventing air from getting to the roots. Hold the plant gently by the stem at soil level and carefully tip it out of the pot. Fill a bowl with lukewarm water, and dip the rootball in, gently rinsing off most of the old soil. Fill a new pot (or the old one, if the plant has not outgrown it) with fresh soil that has been dampened. Replant the rosemary, being careful to layer the roots with the fresh soil and spread them out evenly.

Harvesting and storing: Rosemary can be harvested at any time. To keep the plant healthy, don't take more than 3 to 4 inches off the end of a branch, and never more than 15 percent of the total plant at any one time. Let the trimmed branch dry; then, rub the needles off the rosemary sprig as you would take needles off a Christmas tree. Store the dried needles in a tightly sealed glass container.

Cautions: Do not give rosemary to pregnant cats.

ROSEMARY WASH FOR BALD PATCHES

Adapted from *10 Herbs for Happy, Healthy Dogs,*
by Kathleen Brown (Storey Books, 2000)

This recipe is a quick and easy way to treat abrasions, bites, or any injury that tears the hair away. Rosemary soothes the pain, reduces inflammation, and promotes speedy healing.

> 2 teaspoons rosemary herb
> 1 cup water
> 4 teaspoons witch hazel

To make:
Infuse the rosemary in the water, following the instructions on page 6. Strain, then stir in the witch hazel. Store in the refrigerator, where it will keep for several weeks.

To use:
Saturate a sterile cotton pad with the liquid, and apply to the affected area. Repeat twice a day until new hair growth is well under way.

Valerian
(Valeriana officinalis)

Parts used: Roots

Of historical note: Valerian has had various roles in history. During the Middle Ages, for example, valerian was valued as a spice and as a perfume; during World War I, soldiers relied on the herb to cope with shell shock and battle stress. And interestingly, valerian attracts not only cats but also rats and earthworms.

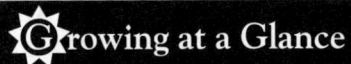

Growing at a Glance

PLANT CYCLE:
Perennial, Zones 4–7

PROPAGATION:
Seed, division

SOIL REQUIREMENTS:
Humus-rich, well drained

LIGHT REQUIREMENTS:
Partial shade

Medicinal uses: Valerian root, a potent natural sedative, smells distinctly like a dirty sock. As unpleasant as this smell is to humans, cats are attracted to it. Valerian functions much like catnip: It is at first stimulating, then sedative. Valerian is extremely helpful in soothing jittery feline nerves, as might occur during a move or when a new pet is introduced to the household. Give ground valerian root in capsule form to your cat, or sprinkle it over your cat's food. You can also offer it in tea or tincture form.

Growing your own: Valerian does best in humus-rich soil; it prefers partial shade but tolerates full sun or full shade. The plant typically reaches 3 to 4 feet in height.

Start seeds indoors in rich soil about eight weeks before the last predicted frost date. The seeds need light to germinate, so cover them with just a dusting of soil at the time of sowing. Keep the soil moist, and make sure the young seedlings receive plenty of sun. Transplant to the garden after the final frost has come and gone. Space plants about 2 feet apart. Valerian can also be propagated by division (see the box on page 22 for instructions).

Harvesting and storing: Harvest valerian roots in the spring or fall of their second year. Wash off the dirt, then place them in a single layer on a tray or cookie sheet. Turn the oven to its lowest setting and put the tray inside, leaving the oven door open an inch or two. The roots are ready when they feel dry and hard (this will take several hours, depending on the size of the roots). Once thoroughly dried, store the roots in a tightly sealed glass container to preserve freshness. Grind the roots only when you're ready to use them.

Cautions: Do not give valerian to pregnant or nursing cats.

VALERIAN FLEA-FREE CAT BED

Your cat will appreciate the calming effects of this valerian-based pillow, as well as enjoy the absence of fleas in bed.

¼ cup ground valerian root
  Pinch ground rosemary
2 tablespoons dill seed
  Thin cushion with a zippered slipcover

Combine the herbs. Distribute the herb mixture in the cushion's slip-cover evenly, making sure that there is a uniform layer beneath the cover, then zip shut. You will need to fluff the pillow every week or so to make sure the herbs are evenly distributed. The herbs should be changed once a month, or when they stop releasing a scent.

Note: To make a more comfortable cat bed, remove some of the cushion's stuffing, making a soft hollow for your cat to lounge in.

Growing Your Own Herbs

Do you love gardening as much as you love your cat? Well, you can combine your affection for both by growing a garden or container pots with cat-friendly herbs.

Garden Paths for Humans and Felines

Paths provide access for plant care and harvesting, especially if the garden is deeper than you can reach. (It's not practical to kneel on the valerian in order to weed the dill.) My favorite paths are made with a series of stepping-stones or neat patterns of slate pieces or bricks. Look for stones that are light in color, so they won't get too hot in the sun, and stones that have a flat surface for sure footing.

As an alternative to paths, you can place large, flat stones in various spots throughout the garden. Place them close enough to-gether that you can get from one to another without stepping in the soil. Make sure that they're big enough to perch on if you'll be using them for weeding access. You might also consider setting a few large, flat black stones in the garden; they'll provide aesthetic effect and offer your cat a warm sunbathing location.

Starting Seeds

Many herb seeds can be sown from seed. Check the herb profiles or the description on the seed packet for information on when to sow them, how deep in the ground to place them, and how much to water them.

Depending on where you live and when winter frosts can be expected to end, you may need to start seeds indoors and transplant the young seedlings outdoors several weeks later. Just follow the steps outlined below.

1. Fill flats or trays with a commercial seed-starting mix. Label each flat with the name of the herb you intend to plant in it.

2. Sprinkle two or three seeds into each cell of the flat.

3. Cover the seeds with a light layer of soil. Check the seed packet to determine how much soil should be used to cover the seeds. Some herbs need only a dusting of soil; others require a light layer of soil.

4. Mist the soil surface with room-temperature water.

5. Cover the flats with plastic wrap, and set them in a warm location that gets plenty of sunlight (or under artificial growing lights).

6. Mist the flats with room-temperature water every day, while checking for seedlings.

7. When seedlings emerge, remove the plastic wrap. Continue to mist daily until it's time to transplant the seedlings to the garden.

8. A couple of weeks before you intend to transplant the seedlings, set them outside in a sheltered location out of direct sunlight for 30 minutes. Then bring them back indoors.

9. On subsequent days, increase the amount of time the plants spend outdoors by 30 minutes.

10. When the plants are acclimated and all risk of frost has passed, transplant the seedlings to the garden. Check the seed packet to determine how far apart the plants should be spaced. For each plant, dig a hole that is twice as wide as and a couple of inches deeper than the container the herb is in. Gently remove the plant from its container and set it in the hole. Fill in the hole with soil, and water well.

Container Gardens

Unfortunately, yard space is not always a luxury that the modern gardener can afford. If you have a patio, deck, or porch or even a well-lit windowsill, however, you have plenty of room for a simple container herb garden. If your container garden is indoors, be sure to keep those plants that are irresistible to cats — namely catnip and valerian — well out of paw's reach.

Containers must have good drainage; be sure that your pots have holes in the bottom to allow excess water to drain out. Container-grown plants need more frequent watering than plants in the ground; check the soil regularly for moisture, and water when it seems dry to the touch. Use a potting mix designed for container plantings; regular soil from your garden is too heavy and will compact, making it difficult for the plants' roots to spread and thrive.

Harvesting and Preserving

With the exception of calendula, which should be harvested in the early afternoon, herbs are most potent when harvested in the morning, after the dew has evaporated. Use clean, sharp scissors to harvest; pinching or pulling at the plants can damage them.

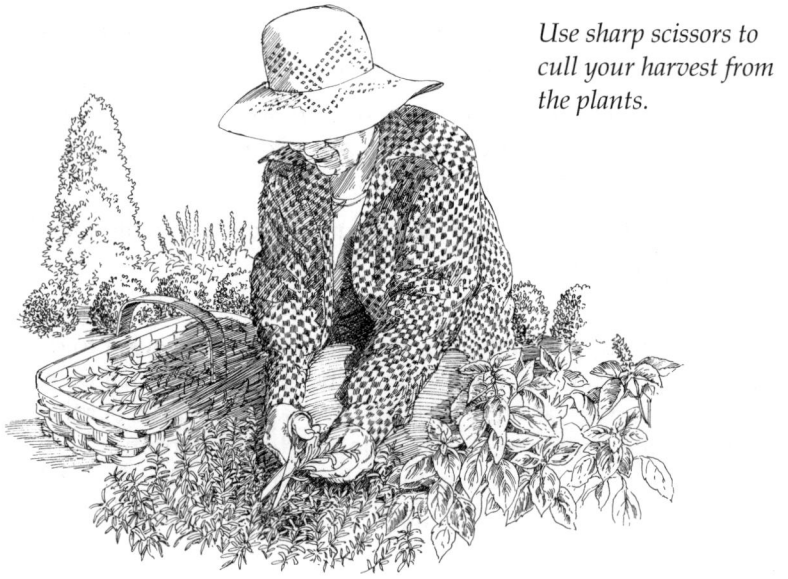

Use sharp scissors to cull your harvest from the plants.

To dry roots, first clean them, then arrange them in a single layer on a cookie sheet or baking tray. Turn your oven to its lowest setting and put the sheet inside, leaving the oven door open an inch or two. When the roots feel dry and hard, they're done. Store them in glass containers in a cool, dark location, where they'll keep for about a year.

To dry leaves and flowers, spread them out in a single layer on a screen. Place the screen in a location that has good air circulation but is not in direct sunlight. Herbs with long stalks can be gathered into bundles and hung upside down. Once they are dry and crackly to the touch, store the herbs in glass containers in a cool, dark location. They'll keep for about a year.

To dry seeds, simply hang the plant stems upside down in a dry location away from direct sunlight. Hang the stems over paper placed on the ground; the seeds will fall from the plants when they are dry. Once the seeds have fallen, you can pick up the paper, bend it into a funnel, and pour the seeds into a container. Or you can place the drying seed heads inside a paper bag, which will catch the seeds as they fall. Poke a few holes in the top of the bag to allow air to circulate. Store seeds in a glass container in a cool, dark location, where they'll keep for about a year.

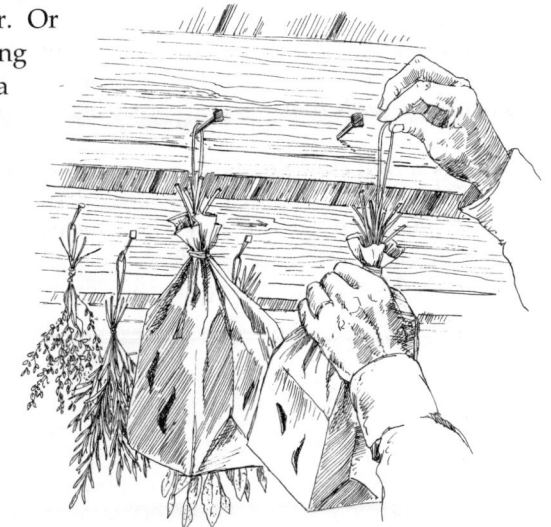

To dry seeds, gather the aerial parts of the herb in bundles. Hang upside down over paper or enclosed in paper bags.

Resources

American Holistic Veterinary Medical Association
410-569-0795
www.ahvma.org
Offers directory of holistic veterinarians as well as directories for the American Academy of Veterinary Homeopathy and the American Academy of Veterinary Acupuncture.

Seed and Gardening Suppliers

Gurney's Seed & Nursery Co.
513-354-1492
www.gurneys.com

Harris Seeds
800-544-7938
www.harrisseeds.com

Johnny's Selected Seeds
877-564-6697
www.johnnyseeds.com

Park Seed Co.
800-845-3369
www.parkseed.com

Pinetree Garden Seeds
207-926-3400
www.superseeds.com

Richter's Herb Specialists
905-640-6677
www.richters.com

Sandy Mush Herb Nursery
828-683-2014
www.sandymushherbs.com

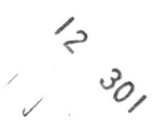